FENG SHUI

FOR 2019

ATTRACT LOTS OF MONEY AND
GOOD LUCK TO YOUR LIFE, HEALTH,
LOVE, ABUNDANCE AND LOTS OF
WEALTH THIS NEW YEAR FOR YOU,
YOUR FAMILY AND YOUR HOME

Jorge O. Chiesa

Table of Contents

Introduction: Getting Started...
What is Feng Shui?

Feng Shui (pronounced fung shway) is an ancient Chinese practice involving art and science. It has existed for thousands of years. The practice is based on the laws of heaven and earth to help people balance their energies within a space. This is to help them receive fortune and health.

The word "feng" means wind and "shui" means water. Therefore, Feng Shui means "wind and water". The local Chinese place the wind that is soft and the water that is clear in one place. It's to represent good health and the harvest.

Feng Shui is proud to think that land includes Chi. Chi work has to do with energy. In ancient times, local Chinese claimed that the earth's energy would be good or bad for others.

Feng Shui comes from Taoist ideals for dealing with nature. Taoism is about religious and philosophical beliefs. Taoism has a strong influence in Asia.

Taoism is also responsible for the birth of the concepts yin and yang. Yin and yang deal with opposite aspects of a phenomenon or compare two phenomena. They represent the quality of correspondence found in most areas of Chinese science and philosophy. An example of this would be ancient Chinese medicine.

In addition to that, the five main elements of Feng Shui are also derived from Feng Shui. When a Feng Shui analysis is done, the compass and Ba-Gua are used. The Ba-Gua is a grid that is created in the shape of an octagon.

This grid has I Ching symbols. In fact, Feng Shui is based on this premise. For you to be able to connect the areas of your home with Feng Shui, you need to understand the concept of Ba-Gua.

The compass is also known as "lo-pan", it works to obtain additional information about an installation. The magnetic needle is surrounded by concentric rings that are strategically placed. The word "it" means everything and "bread" means bowl. Lo-pan is used to open the mysteries of the universe.

When learning Feng Shui, you have to start at the basic level for you to understand the whole process. After you had a good understanding of Feng Shui at the basic level, you will get phenomenal results. The results will affect the way you perceive Feng Shui. You will want to use it regularly in your home and in your business.

When you are committed to Feng Shui, you will need cures to have a better life. There are different things that can be used to accomplish this. Here's five of them:

> Aquarium
> Sources
> Crystals
> Color
> Watches

The methods of Feng Shui

Some of the methods are easy to use; however, when it comes to the main part, it may take some time, such as several years to get used to. Learning Feng Shui is not as easy as people may think it is.

For this type of configuration, you should always start at the beginning with the basics and then move up. It makes it easy for you and others to move forward. Then you can make gradual steps to the advanced phases of Feng Shui. To begin with, here are some things you can implement:

- Air and light of good quality - You must have this in your home to master the principles of Feng Shui. You can benefit from having a good Chi when you incorporate both.

In order to apply this principle, it is a good idea to allow natural light into your home. Windows should be open frequently. If you are a plant lover, invest in some air purifying plants for Feng Shui.

- Ba-Gua - Use the compass to activate the energy map in your house. When you connect to your Ba-Gua, you will discover which areas or rooms of your house are connected to the concept of Feng Shui.

- Get rid of the disorder - You should discard anything that means nothing to you or reminds you of bad events or feelings in your life. If you have a lot of clutter, you can't remove everything overnight.

After doing so, you will feel as if a heavy burden has been lifted from your shoulders. This is a very important thing to do because you will have a release. It will also be easier for you to move on to the next phase.

- **Five Elements** - Familiarize yourself with the five elements of Feng Shui. For certain areas, some elements will have to be stronger. This depends on what you're trying to attract in your life. It also depends on the area of your home you are looking for to implement Feng Shui.

- **Birth Element** - Wood and fire are considered elements and along with that you will need a color to correspond with the elements. In addition to that, you will need to incorporate forms to match the element and color for Feng Shui.

The five elements of Feng Shui

The principle of the five elements is important to the concept of Feng Shui. They work in certain ways according to the rotation of the Productive and Destructive Cycles. The five elements correspond to a certain colour. Some of the elements will use more than one color. The best way to use these elements is to open your space to more happiness.

Here are the five elements and their corresponding colors:

- **Wood** - Represents and provides energy for health and vitality; also represents abundance and is considered a cure for wealth and prosperity. This element resides in the East and Southeast areas of your space. The wood element is also good for use in the south. The colours of the wood element are brown and green.

- **Fire** - Represents high energy and passion; provides energy to things that are related to the race. It will also provide you with assistance in being recognized for your accomplishments. This element resides in the South, Northeast and Southwest areas of your space. The colors of the Fire Element are Red, Orange, Purple, Pink and Strong Yellow.

- **Water** - Represents ease, abundance and freshness; also represents calm and purity. Water represents abundance and is considered a cure for Feng Shui. It can be used in the North, East and Southeast areas of your space. Water Element's colors are blue and black.

- **Earth** - Represents being stable and nourished; also represents the protection of their relationships. It can be used in the Northeast, Southeast and Center areas of your space. The colors of the Earth Element are beige and yellow.

- **Metal** - Represents being precise and clear; it also represents accuracy and efficiency. You can live with clarity and light. It can be used in the West, North and Northwest areas of your space. The Metallic Element is ideal for your home or business. The colours of Metal Element are white and grey.

The Productive and Destructive cycles control the five elements of Feng Shui. The wood forms part of the Productive Cycle that produces the Water Element. The Cycle continues with the creation of Fire, Earth, Metal and last but not least, Water, in that order. The Cycle does not stop and does not complement each other. They also maintain a positive flow between them.

Although it is at the opposite extreme, the Destructive Cycle is as important as the Productive Cycle. Anything that is negative or contributes to decomposition is eliminated. This gives way to things that are positive and will help in the Feng Shui process.

With this Cycle, Wood is responsible for the separation of the Earth. The Earth, in turn, absorbs water; water extinguishes fire; fire melts metal; and metal cuts wood. This is also another cycle that rotates in circles and does not stop.

You will need to use different colors for each direction:

   ✓ *East and Southeast* - Green dominant

   ✓ *South* - Red dominant

   ✓ *Southwest* - Dominant Yellow

   ✓ *West and Northwest* - White or Metallic Dominant

With addresses and color schemes, you

can use alternative colors for the basic ones. Blue and black can be used for east and southeast. Anything from the red family can be used for the southwest and northwest.

Anything from the yellow, beige and brown family, along with any combination, can be used for the West and Northwest. White is the color used in the North because Metal creates Water. In the South, green can be used because Wood creates Fire.

Colors don't have to stand on their own. They can be complemented or combined with others to create powerful statements. With Feng Shui, you must maintain balance and harmony. These attributes are necessary to maintain the flow of Chi in a positive format.

Yang energy comes from the Fire Element. It is represented by the color red.   Other things that help provide more energy are candles and lights. If you want more intimacy when it comes to being close, it would take the Earth's energy. The things that contribute to the earth's energy can help your marriage in a positive way. They can also help you in different relationships.

You can use things like crystals and ceramics, things made of clay to enhance this. Since Metal is created by the Earth, Metal can take advantage of the benefits. Metal is also one of the Yang elements that has a positive effect. Metal is also responsible for creating water. This can help with the flow of Chi.

With water as part of the Chi flow, the flow does not stop. Water helps Chi flow into different areas of life. With Feng Shui, the water that flows is considered calm and relaxing. You can use it to power your home.

If you want to advance or start your professional career, water can be used for that purpose. It also represents wealth and prosperity. A good thing to put into practice for this would be an aquarium or a water source. This can have positive vibrations in certain areas of your home. One place where water is not recommended is the bedroom.

The wood element also connects to your home and garden. Wooden objects can be placed in certain areas to obtain more wealth. They can be placed close to plants and flowers. Another thing that can increase wealth is installing a wooden bench in the area of your garden that is designated for wealth.

The colors of Feng Shui

Black

Black is the color of mystery. It also provides protection. It symbolizes the night when it gets dark and also represents an empty space. Even with that, it provides intensity to any area. If used frequently, it can result in a heavy atmosphere. Black is also used to give strength.

This color can be used in the East, North and Southeast. It should not be used in the South. It can be used in a child's bedroom, but not much. It can also be used in common areas of your home.

If you are trying to attract career opportunities, it can be used in anyone's northern space area. Black can be combined with white for use in furniture.

Brown

The color brown is used in the East, Southeast and South. The energy of this color provides a lot of nutrition. It can be associated with different foods and beverages, such as chocolate and coffee.

Brown can also be used for common areas of your home. You should not wear too much of the color brown for a child's bedroom or southwest area. If there is too much color in an area, it can cause people not to step forward.

Green

This color represents a renaissance and a new beginning. Green provides food and maintains peace in your life. When incorporated with Feng Shui, you should use different green versions, rather than just one.

You can use plants that have fresh foliage. Green is also known to provide healing. It can be used more in the South, East and Southeast zones.

There are different versions of this color that can be used in Feng Shui.

Red

When the colors for Feng Shui are used in the correct format, your environment will be the recipient of good Feng Shui energy. The color red contributes to the Fire Element providing energy.

Fire can be considered a creative and destructive aspect. Fire is a symbol of the sun, of life and of the energy that comes from it. With this Element in your home, you can experience happiness and the desire to become sexually fulfilled.

Red also represents passion and celebration. The Chinese use red for happiness and luck. In India, red is used for marriage and weddings, and in the West, red represents romance and courage.

When people decorate, red is used to enrich themselves. Please note that you should not wear too much red. Otherwise, it can cause anger and excessive stimulation.

With Feng Shui, red can be used in children's rooms with caution. It can also be used in common areas of the house, such as the dining room, living room and kitchen.

In the East, Southeast, West and Northwest areas of your home, you may use the color red, but are limited to the amount you must use. Red is a perfect candidate for use in the South.

Orange

Orange has been dubbed the "social" color. Orange is responsible for providing the energy of Feng Shui to engage in lively conversations and have good feelings in your home. When the winter season is approaching, it can be a reminder of the summer season. Trunk fires also come into play with the color orange.

Just as red represents fire, so does orange. Not a good color for the West and Northwest areas. Besides that, this color should not be seen in the East and Southeast.

These areas are controlled by other elements of Feng Shui.

Orange can be used for common areas such as the living room, dining room, kitchen and anywhere else where the environment can have action and lots of energy. It is a good idea to have some Feng Shui products or accessories.

Since orange is considered a soft and warm color, it is easy to incorporate with Feng Shui. It's a beautiful spectacle to watch as a sunset. It enhances the rooms and makes them stand out.

Purple

Do not abuse the color purple. This color is very strong, and has a relationship with the spirit. Its use on the wall is not recommended. However, it can be used in a space where meditation is taking place. If you use this color at home, be very moderate in your use. You can use lighter colors. It can be used in the East-South and West zones, with limitations.

A good way for the purple color to be implemented is to use Amethyst Feng Shui crystal.

Pink

The color of love is pink. It can also be used to keep energy calm. It also works to calm the heart and give it much love. This color is mainly used in the southwestern area. It's also in line with marriage. When decorating, a soft rose is used. When there is hot and heavy energy, the hot rose is used.

Pink is ideal for use in a little girl's bedroom; what little girl wouldn't want that color? Okay, there may be some, but they're probably few and far between. There are several common pink combinations that include pink and black and pink and green. Pink and green represent activity. Pink and black represent a retro style.

With Feng Shui, rose quartz crystals can be used for love. The crystals are of a soft pink that calms the soul.

Yellow

Yellow is reminiscent of the sun. It can illuminate any space and provide a cozy atmosphere. You have many options to choose from when it comes to yellow. This color is a better choice for a child's bedroom and living room.

If you have a dull looking room, the use of yellow will give you lots of light. Provides the Fire Element, but in a softer format than Red. It's easier to treat on a larger scale. Yellow can also be used to provide self-esteem. If you use hot yellow, don't use too much. Yellow can be used in the Eastern and Southeastern areas.

Grey

Grey is generally considered to be a dull color that doesn't have much life. However, there is a shade of gray (noble gray) that is considered a little more optimistic than the regular color. Gray is used in the western, northwestern, and northern areas of Ba-Gua.

Do not use too much in the East and Southeast. Wood is the dominant element in those areas. Believe it or not, gray can provide Feng Shui energy in most common areas of your home.

It can provide a clear focus to any space in your home. Grey also represents the energy of the Metallic Element.

White

The color white represents the rituals of Yoga. With Feng Shui, it represents tranquility and innocence. It also means beginnings and endings. It has a clean and fresh approach. It can be used for Feng Shui purposes anywhere in your home.

In the East and Southeast, it's not a good idea to use all white. You can use other colors to mix with it.

You may have blank space in your bathroom or in the mediation room. This will help you heal at home. It can also offer possibilities never before explored and a promising future.

Blue

Blue represents clear skies and clear

waters. It can be used in the east and southeast of anyone's space. Since blue is connected to water, energy is responsible for supplying food to the wood element. It can also be used for decoration or art.

Blue can also be used as a color for ceilings. It has been noted that students do better in their studies when they have a blue roof.

For harmony, a light blue color would work well. For peace and quiet, a dark blue color would work better. A deep blue color can be implemented in your bedroom to help you sleep.

For the South, West and Northwest areas, deep blue should not be used much. The colors blue and white can be combined to provide energy.

How to create a happy home with Feng Shui?

Areas that are incorporated with Feng Shui are built to have energy in mind. There is always energy around us that continues to circulate every minute of the day. You can do the same at home. Incorporating the principles of Feng Shui can help you have a healthy and happy home.

When you do this, expect the atmosphere to change. When people come to visit, they will feel happier to be at home and in your presence. When they're happy, you'll be happy. If you were a pessimist before, your behavior will change to the opposite. As long as you keep the positive energy exchange flowing, you will be able to taste the type of environment.

Familiarize yourself with certain areas of your home. The more you are aware of what areas are encompassed, the more successful you will be in incorporating those areas with the principles of Feng Shui. With this, you will be able to transfer it to other areas of your life, including your relationships with family and friends.

Let's look at some things that can move this forward and improve it:

> You must have a connection to your home. Examine the areas of your home and determine which parts are not aligned with the principles of Feng Shui. Anything that is not aligned will eventually have a detrimental effect on your

life. It will also cause you not to have as much energy in those areas.

➢ Don't overreact if your home or the areas in it aren't responding the way you'd like them to. An example would be if you have a basement in your house that needs to be painted, don't bother because it hasn't been painted.

➢ Create some Feng Shui instructions for you so you can go ahead and do the work. Do not get angry or agitated while compiling them. Think of it as something to be done.

➢ There will be a time when you can let your emotions out, but don't let them be an obstacle to your task.

➢ When you eliminate clutter from your home, you are able to provide positive and fresh energy. As a result, your home will also be healthier. Having disorder represents confusion and indecision.

That can turn out to be a negative thing for you if you are working to incorporate Feng Shui into your life. Once the disorder is gone, you'll have a feeling of relief and any stress you've had will be gone. This can also help you have a healthier peace of mind.

Another thing that some people feel they lack is relationships, whether it's a marriage, friendship, or relationship with their children, siblings, parents, or other relatives. How does this work in the equation? Well, having positive relationships can give you more energy.

People want to feel that someone cares about their well-being. Maintaining any type of relationship requires work and does not happen overnight. There are some who are healthy and others who stay on the road.

With respect to your home, there are a few ways that can help you keep your relationships fresh and positive:

- Change the format of your furniture. If you have enough space, move it to another angle or to another wall. Do not store any furniture, such as a sofa, a bed, a table or chairs in the same format each year. It's starting to get monotonous. Moving your furniture can help provide more energy in that area.

- Whatever the area of your home, focus on providing additional energy that is positive. You can do that by eating fresh fruits, fresh flowers, or anything that is fresh and stands out.

- Your bedrooms, bathrooms and closets should be free of clutter. They should be areas that people wouldn't mind seeing if you were showing someone your house.

- Having a TV in your room isn't necessarily a good idea. It can be a distraction from its real purpose.

- Have photos of yourself and your loved ones in a positive format.

- Don't burden people and don't let

them burden you. Everyone needs space and time for themselves.

   - Listen to music that relaxes and calms the soul. Certain types of music can provide great energy in the right environment.

If your home is in chaos... I incorporated Feng Shui as quickly as possible!

Feng Shui may not work too well when your home is located in a cul-de-sac. However, that doesn't speak to all the houses in that curved area. There are some homes that have a good energy flow that still don't get the Chi flow through them.

Here are some explanations as to why a dead end home may not receive the proper flow of Feng Shui it owes:

- When a house is in a dead end, there is a back and forth movement of energy shared between houses of three or more people. The energy within those homes

40

hesitates and cannot be still. This causes less energy to flow; of course, this depends on the houses in that particular cul-de-sac.

Here are some ways to solve the Feng Shui dead end problem:

- The landscape must be clean and provide energy. Houses must also have a quality backing that is robust and enduring. Evergreens can also be installed in the back of the house.

The walkway to the front of the house should be curved. Also in the front of the house, plant some greens and decorate them with colored stones. At least the person who comes to visit you will have something to look at as he walks towards the front of your house.

- Install a fountain or moving water outside your home. Or you could install a bird bath. With Feng Shui, the fountain or bird bath should be installed in the direction in which your home is oriented. In addition, the flow of water must flow in the same direction.

- Your front door may have to be a certain color. If your door is facing north, you can choose a black or blue color for the door. Since that represents calm, you don't have to worry about a lot of confusion in and around your home.

Just remember that every home is different, so there may be some homes within a particular cul-de-sac that may have plenty of power for Feng Shui. There may be some outside that area that don't have that energy. There are several factors involved in this scenario.

Why You Should Not Use Direct Alignment For Your Home Doors

When using Feng Shui, it is important that the doors inside and outside the door are covered. Many people are concerned that this part of the house seems to be in the background. However, it is just as important, if not more important, than the rest of the spaces in the house. Direct alignment of more than one door is not adequate.   It can contribute to evil Feng Shui.

Although the concept of Feng Shui is to have a balance with the flow of energy in your home, having a direct alignment with more than one door cannot work. The quality of Feng Shui power flow is subject to decrease.

One area where you don't want to do this is with the front and back doors. Most of the energy of good Feng Shui comes from the front door. If those two doors are aligned, energy can travel through the back door. This is not good because the energy of good Feng Shui needs to penetrate through your home. Food is also necessary.

Take note of the type of energy being created in your home. If that's not enough, see what you can do to create more energy for better Feng Shui. However, if your door has doors in your home that are directly aligned with each other, there are some things you can do to remedy that situation:

- In order for you to be able to change the way the doors are located, you may need to change the color of one of the doors. After the color change, the relationship will be different, one of the doors will have more strength than the other.

- Where the energy is, you can put a little round table there. The energy will be directed elsewhere and the energy will slow down. To improve, add a vase or similar container with fresh flowers. Doing this will give more credibility to the energy.

- If you don't want to use fresh flowers, get a plant with a pot. Having a plant will also send power in another direction.

The purpose of doing these things is to

redirect the energy in another direction. Don't forget to incorporate Chi and send the water flow in another direction. It is important to keep the energy of Feng Shui flowing in your home.

Feng Shui for your kitchen

Incorporating Feng Shui into your kitchen will take some time. You have to see how it is placed inside the house. The kitchen is usually located next to the backyard of the house. There's a good reason for that.

From a visual point of view, if the kitchen was near or in the front, it could pose a mentality of problems with food and nutrition. Having it in the front of the house can mean that you may be tempted to eat every time it comes in. It would be just as bad if you had guests coming to visit us. The first thing they'd like to do is eat.

However, if your home is configured this

way, you can do something about it. You can buy a curtain and install it in the kitchen entrance area. Or, you could measure the French doors to install in that area. Another idea that you could implement is to have something that arouses your interest. This can cause a distraction in the real focus (the kitchen).

If you are cooking, you should have an eye on the kitchen entrance. There's a kitchen where the stove faces the wall. To implement the Feng Shui method, people who are cooking can put a mirror on the stove.

For newer homes, builders are now including islands that are in the center of the kitchen area. This would be a good addition to the concept of Feng Shui. When the island is strategically located in the center, the person cooking can see what is happening in another area.

When set up in this way, they can continue to participate in what is happening in a nearby area, in addition to continuing to cook.

This type of kitchen configuration is attractive because it allows other people to come in and help cook. The original person who was cooking won't feel underappreciated. It can contribute to greater camaraderie and bonding in relationships.

In Feng Shui, the stove is the symbol of health and wealth. All burners must be used equally in rotation. Do not use one or two burners and leave the rest unused. Using all four in an equal rotation can cause you to receive money from more than one source.

It has been noted that with older stoves, these are really better because they incorporate the Feng Shui method to reduce speed. Take a good look at what's going on and what you're doing.

Although microwave-cooked foods can be quick and convenient, you may feel rushed in the meantime.   People who faithfully practice the Feng Shui method do not like to use microwaves because of the large amount of radiation.

The kitchen should be one of the cleanest areas of the house. It must also be free of disorder. If you have something that isn't working properly or isn't working at all, you should discard it. Having something that doesn't work or doesn't work properly is contrary to the purpose and principles of Feng Shui.

You can also use different methods and design patterns of the Feng Shui concept. The most commonly used methods are a Shaker style concept, contemporary with solid colors and wood grain and a rich look that comes with carvings and other related items.

The kitchen must have adequate lighting and use different types. There must be enough room to move. The more space you have, the better. If this means you have to move machines and appliances to create more space, so be it.

You don't need much kitchen equipment or utensils in front of you. Use only the things you're going to cook with. When you're done with those items, you can place them in the sink for later washing. At least they'll be out of the way.

To increase energy in the kitchen, you may want to have some fruit, flowers or a plant on the table. This will also make the kitchen look more attractive. Cooking in the kitchen is where the heart is. You want to have a place where people can come and enjoy your company.

Create wealth and abundance by using Feng Shui in your bathroom

A bath is one of the places where you can incorporate Feng Shui for wealth purposes. There are different strategies you can use to achieve this.

- Color - From the different elements, you can use different colors to achieve your goal of attracting abundance from using Feng Shui. With Wood, brown and green should be used; with Water, blue and black; with Earth, colors from the yellow and brown collection can be used, such as light yellow or light beige.

- Crystals - You can buy Feng Shui crystals to use. Mix them with amethyst, citrine, rose quartz and others from the crystal family. This combination can create an abundance cure in Feng Shui.

- Bamboo - Another Feng Shui cure for wealth and abundance is to have 8 stems of Lucky Bamboo. This cure is used by many people and can be found in many flower retailers.

On the other hand, there are people who don't take care of them as they should. Bamboo is very easy to maintain, but people don't try hard to do it. It represents tranquility and relaxation. The five elements of Feng Shui have a role to play in the bamboo plant.

- Atmosphere - Decorate your bathroom to make it look like a spa. A spa is a place where you can relax. Getting a massage will take all the worries out of the world. All you'll ever think about is peace of mind.

- Disorder - Eliminate any excess or disorder that does not need to be there. If you have items that have expired, get rid of them. If there are things you haven't used in a long time, get rid of them too. You want to have things in your bathroom that represent positive energy. It is also important that the lighting is good.

- Meaning of Wealth - Whatever wealth it means to you, put it in the bathroom. It can be a photo, a poem or a quote that reminds you of wealth.

- Toilet Seat - Toilet seat must remain down when not in use. This will demonstrate that the energy will be maintained and not spread everywhere outside that area.

Implementation of mirrors with the concept of Feng Shui

Mirrors are generally used as a reflection. People use them to look at themselves. With Feng Shui, they help bring water. They are also used to attract the Chi method in addition to expanding the space. Mirrors can change the way energy flows in a given area. They are good for bringing peace and a new perspective on life.

With Feng Shui, three types of mirrors are used. Here is a brief synopsis of them:

➢ **Convex** - These mirrors are considered to represent protection. They are the eyes and ears and most of the time, are used apart from Feng Shui. They can also be used within the concept, but they have to be framed in a certain way.

➤ **Concaves** - Most of the time, these mirrors are not used within Feng Shui. The reflection of the mirrors is a smaller version that is turned upside down.

➤ **Typical** - Depending on the shape and frame, it represents some Feng Shui healing. They are usually placed in the southwestern part of your area.

There is also the Ba-Gua mirror, which is separate from the three mirrors mentioned above. It's very powerful and for the most part, people don't use it properly. It's only made for exteriors, not interiors. If you are not feeling the right energy in your home or business, then this type of mirror will be useful to you. This mirror should not be used for decoration.

The Ba-Gua mirror is available in concave and convex formats. Ba-Gua is made of wood and you can choose between green, red or gold.

The Ba-Gua mirror is good to use if you need to protect yourself from harm or danger, such as attacks against you or if there are people who want to hurt you.

You should consult with a well-informed Feng Shui person to place you in the correct area. Most of the time, it is placed above the main entrance of your home. One place not to be placed is in the living room.

Feng Shui in your bedroom to enhance your love life

To have a positive and intimate relationship with your partner, you need a good feng shui room. Both will be able to spend time renewing themselves, without having to deal with many unnecessary things.

Only one important piece of furniture should be placed in your bedroom and that is the bed. You have to have something to sleep on. Get something simple like a wooden bed frame along with a natural mattress. The sheets under which you sleep should be made of the best quality cotton or fence. It doesn't have any electronics except things like a clock.

Part of Yin culture includes sleeping. It is important that the bedroom is located in the back of your house, where activity is minimal. Your bedroom should look warm and cozy. After all, it's where you share intimate, tender moments alone.

Here are some more Feng Shui suggestions that you can use for your bedroom:

- The bedroom should not be placed over the garage. This is where you can incorporate low energy and problems with your health. In addition, the electrical elements of the vehicle parked in the garage can interfere with your electromagnetic system.

- Try not to use electrically powered items in the bedroom. These items can cause a high electrical charge.

- If possible, the bedroom should not be anywhere in the children's kitchen, bathroom, living room or bedroom.

- To keep the flames burning in your sex and love life, there must always be fresh energy in the bedroom. This can be implemented using crystals, candles or essential oils.

Keeping the bedroom with a good Feng Shui will help maintain a positive flow and sensual feelings of energy. A good Feng Shui bedroom should be filled with lots of love and passion. It should also be exciting and provide relaxation.

Here are a few more ways you can create a good Feng Shui bedroom:

- Don't have stale air in your room. Open the window and let in some fresh air, weather permitting. You should have fresh air flowing into your bedroom. In addition to eliminating most appliances, it is also not advisable to have plants in the bedroom.

- The lighting in the bedroom must be adjustable. The easiest way to do this is to install an attenuation switch. You can adjust the lights to an appropriate level. You can also use candles, but buy candles that do not contain toxins.

Use colors that correspond to the Feng Shui method. Colors should create a balance for the bedroom. In this way, you will be assured of a positive energy flow. This will help you sleep better. It will also help your sex life. Some colors that would work well in the bedroom are white and chocolate brown.

If you want to add art to your bedroom, choose pieces that reflect how you see your life and your future in a positive way. Do not use parts that represent anything to the contrary.

The Feng Shui procedure for your bed should be as follows: You should be able to access your bed from both sides. The bed must not be parallel to the bedroom door. You can have two small tables on either side of the bed. Doing these things will help your bed and bedroom balance.

All doors that are connected to the bedroom must be closed. Whether it's the front door, the cabinet door or the inside bathroom door, none of them should be ajar. This will keep the energy flow inside the bedroom. It will also improve your relationship with your partner.

You want to have a bedroom that will be the symbol of pleasure, intimacy and love. Using the Feng Shui method can help you do exactly that.

Your business at home, thanks to Feng Shui

Believe it or not, there are many business people all over the world who use the principles of Feng Shui in their business. Many Asians believe that Feng Shui is necessary for proper business management. In fact, there are some famous entrepreneurs in the United States who are using Feng Shui and have found good success in their business.

Many people have become entrepreneurs and have established their office at home. This is a cost-effective way to start because there aren't many overheads.

On the other hand, some people who

work from home find themselves somewhat perplexed because it can be difficult for them to separate their home business from their personal life and they don't have much interaction with other people. However, having a home-based business overcomes the challenges and frustrations people face when working in a 9 to 5 year job.

If you are looking to attract wealth and wealth for your home-based business using Feng Shui, here are some ways to incorporate it:

- ✓ You should always sit with a solid wall behind your back. Avoid sitting with a window behind you.

- ✓ You should not have a wall in front of you while you are at your desk working or when you enter the office.

✓ Wherever your wealth area is, you should have office equipment there.

✓ For Chi to flow harmoniously, place tables and chairs in a strategic format.

✓ Have air purifying plants in your home office. This will help provide you with fresh air quality and will also increase the amount of oxygen generated in that area.

✓ Apart from air-purifying plants, refrain from having plants with sharp edges, such as cactus.

✓ The front door to your home office should be free of obstructions. If there is an obstruction, such as a table behind the door, the Chi will not function properly.

✓ To increase the presence of Chi, a good idea is to install a hanging glass in your home office.

✓ Your home office should be a good distance from your bedroom.

✓ Your home office should be about productivity. The colors of your home office should reflect that.

✓ The photocopier should not be near the main entrance door. The heat from the photocopier may cause the Chi not to flow properly.

✓ If there is an empty vase near the main entrance door, Chi will find its way into the empty vase. This will harm the environment.

✓ If you have clients who come to see you, try placing a fish tank within the wealth area. This will help you get better results and probably more customers, which in turn means more money. You have to be careful to follow the instructions to do this, otherwise it won't work.

✓ For Chi to work properly, install a small indoor fountain in the wealth corner. This method will also help your health.

✓ Keep your desks and surrounding areas free of clutter. To help with this, the Chinese don't use paper trays. The concept is beginning to make its way into the United States.

✓ Pay attention to the type of light you are using in your home office. You must use both natural and artificial lighting. It won't work properly if you don't have enough natural light.

You should also think about getting other types of lights, such as full spectrum lights. These lights are similar to the natural light spectrum and have been rated healthier to use.

There are different areas of your home office that need to be nurtured with Feng Shui. In the North zone, in addition to Metal, the Water Element is used. In your home office, it's okay to have images with black and white frames.

The southern zone uses fire as a source of energy. You should refrain from having blue mirrors or images of water representing this color. The southeastern area is for images that represent prosperity and abundance. The wood element is used here. With this, you should refrain from images of Fire and Metal.

Using these Feng Shui principles will help your business prosper and grow in prosperity and abundance.

Use Feng Shui for Your Internet Business

You can use Feng Shui to create harmony for your websites. Your web pages must be aligned correctly. You want visitors who come to your site to have easy navigation and access. It should be a positive experience for them.

Pages should be clean and use bright colors for the background. If you create web pages with a dark color, it can be a nuisance for those who are visiting your website. To start the Chi flow, you can use bold colors.

White and blue are some of the ones that come to mind. These colors are the symbols of air and water. If you use colors that don't mix very well, your website won't be attractive. You can incorporate evil Feng Shui if it doesn't look good.

Refrain from adding things like animated graphics that remove the essence of the website. If it has to be part of the website, then make sure it is something that looks natural.

On your website, you must have an area that displays a logo. This logo will be on every web page you create. Refrain from putting many games and other tricks on your website and web pages. This may distract visitors.

Your website must have a main menu page. All the elements you are putting on the website should not be lined up on one side of the screen or cluttered on both sides of the screen.

Don't make your website look so professional that no one wants to stay. Create websites that bring harmony and good atmosphere to visitors. If you are going to incorporate music, use music that is relaxing. This will help to create a positive Chi.

The important thing with creating websites using Feng Shui is that you want them to be simple, easy to navigate and not look rushed or messy. Too many things in it and people will turn around in the blink of an eye.

Ironically, having a rushed or messy website can be a reflection of the person themselves. It's about having a positive flow so the good Chi continues to flow.

Using Feng Shui for a Retail Business

You may want to open a retail store. You have many products, but you have no idea how to attract or keep customers once they have set foot in your business. You don't understand what's going on and you need help in this field.

Using the principles of Feng Shui can change your situation. Here are some things you can do to change the atmosphere of your business:

- You've got too many things piled up. The products are nice, but there's no sense of what goes where. Or they may be thinking, "Why is this product here when it should be somewhere else?"

You must remove some of the products and leave some space between them. Grouping them together only causes confusion for the client. They feel it's too much for them to see.

Try to put the products in different categories.   Then you'll see the difference when the customers come in. They will want to stay longer and watch because they are not confused or frustrated with what they are going to buy.

- Feng Shui energy from the front door to the back door does not flow properly. In turn, you don't get customers or sales. The moment the customer walks through the door, he needs to be attracted by what you have.

Be clear about the products you offer and their benefits. Customers always want to know what they're getting out of it. After all, you're promoting them, so why don't you let them know how they can benefit from buying?

The driveway and front area should be more visible than the back. They'll see the front of the store first before they come back.

- Your halls aren't clear. You have things on the road that are creating obstacles for the customer. It shouldn't be like that. A customer doesn't want to be squeezing or stepping on things just to get ahead. Make room in the aisles for easy access to products.

Some of these suggestions can also be implemented for the Internet. Take a survey or ask some of your customers if there are things you can make changes in your store. You might be surprised with the answers. It is very important that you adapt to the needs of the client. Without them, there'd be no business.

How to get a Feng Shui consultant?

There are many people who are not sure what to do first when it comes to Feng Shui. They may need more information to make a decision about whether this is for them or not. If you need the services of a Feng Shui consultant, investigate very carefully and thoroughly.

You can probably get more information online and keep going from there. Write down everything you want from the consultant. There are also some schools where Feng Shui is taught.

You may want to check there to find someone who can help you. You can also ask people you know if they have any recommendations. You never know who else has gone through this process.

Once you come up with some names, interview them and check their backgrounds. Don't be afraid to ask for references. They should be more than willing to provide you with this information. Let them know what you're looking for. Once you've solved it, you can check which one best suits your needs.

Conclusion

Whether it's to improve your health, your love life or your finances, Feng Shui has been incorporated as a way to do it. The method has worked for the Chinese people for many years. Since it has spread, people have been curious to know how you can help them. This e-book has provided much information to begin your journey into abundance and other things that can improve your life.

If you stay on the right track with this and are serious about making significant changes in your life, you will see a difference. You'll be surprised how healthy you've become. You'll be so excited to be intimate with your partner that it'll take your breath away. With your finances, you can have more money than you once dreamed possible when using the Feng Shui method.

Just remember that everything will not happen overnight and that it will take time before you see a change in your life for the better.

Now yes, I wish you the best in your results, and remember, everything is practical; theory without action is of no use to you. It brings everything you learn into real life.

A big hug, your friend, Jorge!

By the way, when you achieve your results little by little, I highly recommend you, if you want to improve your social skills, my book "HOW TO CONTROL SOCIAL ANSIEDAD AND PANIC ATTACKS", is a book that I am sure will help you a lot to avoid any kind of anxiety. Without further ado, you can find it in the Amazon search engine, like: "How to control social anxiety and panic attacks" or searching for my name "Jorge O. Chiesa"... Once again I wish you success in your results!

Printed in Poland
by Amazon Fulfillment
Poland Sp. z o.o., Wrocław